An Introduction to
Living Well with Pain

Frances Cole

ROBINSON

ROBINSON

First published in Great Britain in 2017 by Robinson

1 3 5 7 9 10 8 6 4 2

A CIP catalogue record for this book
is available from the British Library.

Footprint illustration © iStock
Thoughts image on page 24 © Marrio31/iStock
Images copyright © Liane Payne on pages xii, xiv, 26, 67, 106 and 107
All other images copyright © David Andrassy

Important note
This book is not intended as a substitute for medical advice or
treatment. Any person with a condition requiring medical
attention should consult a qualified medical practitioner
or suitable therapist.

ISBN: 978-1-47213-771-5

Typeset in Bembo by Initial Typesetting Services, Edinburgh
Printed and bound in Great Britain by CPI Group (UK) Ltd

Papers used by Robinson are from well-managed forests
and other responsible sources.

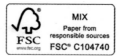

Robinson
An imprint of
Little, Brown Book Group
Carmelite House
50 Victoria Embankment
London EC4Y 0DZ

An Hachette UK Company
www.hachette.co.uk
www.littlebrown.co.uk

Living Well with Pain

Contents

Acknowledgements   vii

Introduction   ix

Footstep 1: What do we know about
            persistent pain?   1

Footstep 2: Acceptance   9

Footstep 3: Pacing every day for better times   17

Footstep 4: Set goals, action plans and rewards   28

Footstep 5: Getting fit and staying active   40

Footstep 6: Managing moods   50

Footstep 7: Sleep well more often   64

Footstep 8: Healthy eating, managing
            relationships and coping with work   76

Footstep 9: Relaxation and mindfulness:
            Soothe the body and mind   85

Footstep 10: Managing setbacks   96

Appendices   105

Resources   110

For Chris, whose courage and compassion
are inspirational

Acknowledgements

This book emerged with the help of many people with pain and I wish to thank them, including Pete Moore (www.paintoolkit.org). Pete kindly shared much of his self-management experience to ensure we have captured the struggles and successes of living well with pain – not an easy task.

I am very grateful to numerous colleagues in pain management, who enabled the book to emerge. Zoe Malpus provided a compilation of insights from people with pain and their views of compassion that shaped the book in places. Stanter Kandola gave her experience and insights of both personal pain and mindfulness. Polly Ashworth guided the content on sleep with valuable resourced materials.

I am very grateful to several people who helped with the content in editing and suggesting useful changes. Nicola Sternberg helped make it happen, rapidly responding to author's needs, and Lorna Fenton did a sterling job of ensuring readability and content. Judith Hooper provided valuable feedback and suggested amendments at the final stages. Andrew McAleer at Little, Brown Book Group was both most supportive and encouraging as deadlines slipped.

I hope it proves a valued resource to guide many with pain to build resilience, new lives and overcome losses. Living well with pain can be an incredible journey of change which has rich rewards and knotty unresolved problems that become easier to bear with kindness and care to oneself.

My reward for the effort and success of reaching this goal is a new bicycle!

Frances Cole

Introduction

Living with persistent pain is distressing, confusing and exhausting. Treatments only help some, and may even add to the challenge of living with pain. There are other ways to take control of your pain and day-to-day life. People with pain find that learning ways to manage pain and regain their life makes a huge positive difference to them and others. This book has ten Footsteps to explore and learn those skills to grow in confidence in self-managing pain with kindness.

Our life journey can change direction often for all sorts of reasons and usually we are in charge of those changes. However, when persistent pain arrives it can take over and leave us feeling out of control. We can find ourselves on a very different journey and this can feel quite scary.

People with pain have shared that not knowing how to manage their pain was just as frustrating as trying to find ways to get it fixed. Learning to cope well with pain made a valued difference:

'I'm getting a life back; better at accepting the changes now'

'I've learnt self-compassion and how to take time out from my day for myself'

'I've broken the circle of pain and slowly found that exercise actually reduces pain'

'I have far greater control over the pain and do not always depend on tablets'

An Introduction to Living Well with Pain will guide you along your self-management journey. Like a kind and patient friend, it can support you to take footsteps in the right direction so that you get your life on track. Pain is isolating. It makes you feel different, unconnected to others and very judgemental of yourself and sometimes others too. This book draws on different areas of pain management including talking therapies such as Cognitive Behavioural Therapy (CBT), Acceptance and Commitment Therapy (ACT) and Compassion Focused Therapy (CFT), fitness coaching and mindfulness training. It shares the true stories, experiences and wisdom of people with pain (although names have been changed to protect anonymity).

Use the guide to build your confidence and find balanced ways of living well with pain. You could set yourself the target of trying one new Footstep each week or you could focus on one Footstep now, adding others at a later date. Change can take time and day by day you will find that you become better and better at putting into practice the skills and ideas in this book. Expect to work steadily for some weeks or months until you find that skills like balancing activities or setting goals are another everyday routine.

Resources and help are suggested with each Footstep. In some Footsteps, Pete Moore of the Pain Toolkit (www.paintoolkit.org) shares his experience of living well with pain to guide progress. There are links to trusted videos, books and websites to discover more about self-management from people with pain and professionals. The Footsteps do not explore in detail any medical treatments, as their focus is on self-management. Pain management programmes, either group or on-line course options, can offer additional skills and learning and grow confidence further.

Where to start on the first footsteps?

First action: let's explore these two circles to guide your journey to living well with pain. First look at the **Pain circle** overleaf which shows how your pain traps you in this vicious circle. Put a ring around the struggles that affect you now, day to day.

PAIN CIRCLE

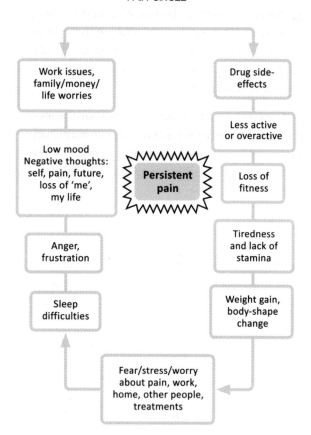

Second action: Explore the **Living my life well circle** overleaf with its Footsteps of skills and ways to break out of the pain circle. Choose **three areas** that you want to take action on <u>**now**</u> to decrease your day-to-day struggles. This will guide you to the Footstep/s to start on.

Still unsure or stuck? People with pain say the most valued Footsteps are acceptance, pacing and managing moods, and being patient with yourself! These ideas may help you to get going and, wherever you start, good luck.

Living-my-life-well circle

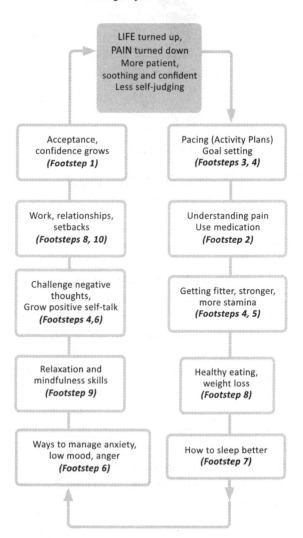

LIFE turned up,
PAIN turned down
More patient,
soothing and confident
Less self-judging

Acceptance,
confidence grows
(Footstep 1)

Pacing (Activity Plans)
Goal setting
(Footsteps 3, 4)

Work, relationships,
setbacks
(Footsteps 8, 10)

Understanding pain
Use medication
(Footstep 2)

Challenge negative
thoughts,
Grow positive self-talk
(Footsteps 4,6)

Getting fitter, stronger,
more stamina
(Footsteps 4, 5)

Relaxation and
mindfulness skills
(Footstep 9)

Healthy eating,
weight loss
(Footstep 8)

Ways to manage anxiety,
low mood, anger
(Footstep 6)

How to sleep better
(Footstep 7)

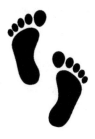

Footstep 1:

What do we know about persistent pain?

Persistent pain, sometimes known as chronic pain, is pain that continues for three months or more after healing has occurred. Persistent pain happens because the body is unable to switch the pain sensations off in the nervous system, including within the brain. Such sensations can resemble the original injury or damage, so it feels as though the damage has not healed, when it actually has. The original cause may be obvious, such as shingles which is a viral infection that damages a nerve which sets off pain sensations. Other causes might be trauma or a long-term illness such as diabetic neuropathy or the after-effects of a stroke. Sometimes the cause is not obvious and the problems are within the pain system itself.

It leaves the millions of people with persistent pain frustrated, as they feel something is still wrong in their body – so why can't it be fixed? This leads them to search for a cure (like Pete Moore's story in Footstep 2). Sadly, the pain sensations have become permanent. Persistent pain is like a radio that is switched on permanently with the volume turned up. So what can change? It is possible to turn the volume down but realise and accept that the noisy radio cannot be switched off completely.

What is pain?

Pain is felt when the brain picks up messages of harm or danger to the body. Nerve endings are sensors designed to notice changes like touch and pressure, or hot or cold temperatures that can harm or danger to the body.

It is helpful to think of mind and brain as having different roles or jobs to do:

- Your mind deals with your thinking – like memories, images, words, beliefs and feelings or emotions – and a range of physical sensations – like smell, taste, touch, sound.

- Your brain is the physical structure that is the control centre for the whole body via the nervous system and other systems.

Key message: pain helps the brain protect itself and the body too

Nerve-ending sensors send chemical and electrical messages through nerves and the spinal cord to alert the brain continuously and especially if there is danger to it or the body. The brain, with the mind, deals with all this information and quickly decides how to react to reduce the danger. They react by checking many, many areas within the brain and body at the same time. For example, if you twisted your wrist opening a tight jar your brain and mind check things such as:

- **Memories** of previous injuries in this area of the body: 'The last time it felt like this I had tripped and broken my wrist and it really hurt'. These memories are often in pictures in the mind, so can be vivid and alarming, making you feel scared – this fear makes your pain system more sensitive.

- **Location of pain**: 'Where is the pain now? What sort of pain is it? Is it coming from tissues like skin, muscle, tendons, joints or structures like lungs, stomach, and bladder, etc.?' The brain checks the system, just like an airline pilot checks the different flight deck displays to ensure the plane systems are all working correctly. If there is a fault or alarm in one, then takes action to keep the plane safe. The brain does this automatically and without you being aware.

- **Focus of attention** of the brain: assessing, 'Is this pain worth focusing on now as I am busy watching an exciting movie or cooking dinner or doing . . . ' This guides **action to protect the wrist:** 'Shall I move it or shall I freeze so as not to injure my wrist any further?'

- **Feeling anxious and with thoughts about the pain:** 'I cannot move it, it must be broken again . . . ' so fear and panic set in and this increases the sensitivity of the pain networks in the nerves and brain.

- **Identifying the pain cause itself:** 'Is this a fracture? Is this a strained muscle? Is it a friction burn or a bruise?'

All this brain and mind activity happens without us being aware of most of it, and very quickly.

Pain protects you

Touching a hot dish by accident makes the nerve sensors send signals through the nerves (similar to electrical wires) straight to your spinal cord and your brain. Within milliseconds your hand moves away as your brain has registered danger and damage to the skin and flesh. The acute pain protects you. Acute pain happens for many reasons; infections like tonsillitis, injury, a fractured bone, damage to nerves like a slipped spinal disc. If areas are damaged then, as they heal, the pain reduces and disappears in around three months.

Pain becoming persistent

'It still hurts me' . . . even after three months of healing and repair time. This means it is likely to be persistent pain. It is linked not to one problem or fault in the nervous system, rather to many different problems in many places in the nervous system and the brain such as:

1. More sensitivity in the sensors to pressure, touch, heat or cold in the skin or in tissues like muscle, or in nerves themselves, or in the organs like the stomach or kidneys.

2. Nerves themselves, if damaged by pressure, disease, infection or trauma, become more excitable; so slight pressure causes lots of painful electrical shocks or unpleasant sensations like pins and needles. Shingles is an example of nerve damage due to infection.

3. The brain has systems that can turn pain down or switch it off, like a brake to slow or stop a car. In persistent pain, this brake activity in the brain is faulty as the supply of nerve transmission chemicals becomes run down.

Pain is very isolating and invisible, so no one else sees or feels the pain. This adds to the frustration of living with it. Emotions like anger and anxiety can wind up pain nerve networks, making them more sensitive; remember, this is not your fault.

So what can you do to reduce persistent pain?

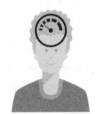

Help your brain
turn down the pain

The most effective way of reducing pain is *changing the way you think* and managing your pain. It can come as a bit of shock to realise that, to reduce your pain means that *you* need to help your mind and brain to turn the pain down. Retraining them means helping them become more aware the body is getting fitter and stronger, daily activities are balanced and your mind is more goal-focused, less pain-focused. Retraining them is helped by:

- Focusing on soothing in different ways, like breathing to relax or listening to calming music.

- Practising being supportive and caring to yourself, as this helps wind down the sensitive pain system. So, in a sense, it helps the brain reduce the volume on the noisy radio, tuning out some of the pain.

Then slowly over weeks and months, the brain learns you are living a more healthy life, being more active, doing things normally, focusing on living well and feeling less stressed by pain itself.

So we cannot fix persistent pain. People can reduce some pain themselves by building their own confident future through self-management and their best treatment options. These treatment options can be medications or devices. Some people find using little or no medication is better. It is a tricky balance. This book will help you learn those skills and techniques to manage your pain and your life better, *so that you run your life rather than letting the pain run you.* Explore the video examples in the resources section to understand much more about pain.

Persistent pain and medication

Managing persistent pain with medication can be helpful in shrinking pain. But equally it may have side effects (possibly harmful and unpleasant ones) and may not work well in the long term. Strong opioids such as codeine, tramadol, oxycodone and morphine have considerable side effects including dependency or addiction. Only a very few people with persistent pain are helped by them. So try them for up to no more than around eight to twelve weeks, with regular reviews with your clinician on their benefits/side effects. If there are no real benefits that help you to self-manage better and achieve your personal goals, then reduce and stop them. Long term, people choose to stop them if they get poor pain relief and suffer harmful side effects. Check the resources for more information.

Working with a clinician who understands pain and medication is important. A trial of medication with regular reviews is useful to see if it helps you achieve your action plans and goals (see Footstep 4: Set goals, action plans and rewards). If you take long-term medication, a six-monthly or annual review with your clinician is vital along with sharing your action plans and goals. This is just like having a regular dental check-up.

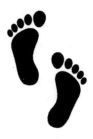

Footstep 2:

Acceptance

People with pain find it helps hugely to accept persistent pain as part of their day-to-day life. The constant struggle to avoid or reduce pain can be very stressful. Learning to observe, understand and accept persistent pain allows you to gain control over your life.

Donna's Acceptance Story

Donna found that acceptance didn't happen overnight. It was something she learnt to do over time:

'You don't just suddenly wake up and go, "I've accepted my pain." It's a long journey you're on and the road is twisty and you can come off it now and then. It was a gradual thing – I can't tell you the day I accepted I would always have persistent pain, but I knew I'd got there when I was no longer battling with my body.'

So what do we mean by acceptance?

It is hard to accept that pain will not shrink away from your life. Acceptance means being willing to take steps to move on, despite the pain. It is about shifting your attention from what you can't change – the pain – to what you can change. Pete Moore, from the Pain Toolkit (www.paintoolkit.org) shares what acceptance meant for him.

Pete's acceptance story

Accepting that pain was going to be with me for the rest of my life was a real tough hurdle. Before I got to the point of acceptance I did everything I could do to get rid of the pain. I kept seeing the doctor and I spent around £24,000 on consultations and treatments with people who I hoped would take my pain away. It all failed and I was £24,000 worse off. I still had pain and felt pretty depressed.

I had to surrender to the fact that I would have some sort of pain for the rest of my life. So the bigger question was, 'What could I do about it?' I didn't have the skills or the confidence to work this out myself. I needed help, fast.

I was lucky to get a place on a Pain Management Programme (PMP) in London, sadly with an eighteen-month waiting list. So I had to learn patience as well! The PMP gave me the skills, and more crucially, the confidence, to manage my pain myself, and get my life back on track.

It seems that people with pain need to get to the point of acceptance in their own way, and in their own time. All I can say is that for me, it was only when I accepted my lot with my pain that the doors of help and support opened. Life turned a positive corner and I could change and control many things in my life again.

Why is acceptance important?

Often, waiting for healthcare teams or specialists to explain and fix your pain can lead to feelings of frustration and stress. Many people with pain are stuck in this turmoil. It's normal, because our human brains tend to focus on trying to *fix a problem* rather than looking for helpful ways to *live with it*. Many people have found, by trial and error, the way forward is to be more accepting.

This is not easy and it is certainly not about giving in or resigning yourself to pain. It can be hard to accept you are not the person you were and that your life is different now. However, if you can accept things have changed, then you can switch your focus and energy to living well. Your day-to-day life will be led by your plans and ideas of what is possible, not the pain. You can plan and run each day in a different way and at the right speed. You can experiment and learn all the time, and use action plans and goals to keep on track.

This is self-management. The Footsteps in this guide will help you learn the skills that you need, including how to pace yourself, set goals and manage your moods. Setbacks are to be expected and this guide will help you find ways to cope with difficulties when they come up.

What helps to be more accepting?

Focus on what you can change

Many people with pain have been on long journeys to try and answer the 'Why pain?' question. They have spent a lot of time and (like Pete Moore) possibly a lot of money seeking an explanation and solution for their pain. Sadly, it is not always possible for persistent pain to be cured or fixed. We now understand a lot more about pain, the brain and pain nerve networks. We know that to remove persistent pain permanently, by searching for and fixing the problem/s, is an impossible task. In fact, often people find that when they focus on their pain and try to solve it, their pain systems actually become more sensitive. Explore Footstep 1, about persistent pain, and its links, to discover more about pain systems.

Self-managing pain means choosing to pause, think and use skills and resources to cope better. Then add trial and error to discover what works well for you most of the time.

Ways to help with acceptance

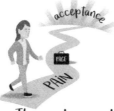

The winding road
to acceptance

Acceptance is not something that happens over-night.

It can be about:

- slowly adjusting how you do things

- accepting and adapting to being a different person

- thinking and viewing yourself and life differently

- patiently and steadily shifting the focus to what you really want to do each day

- shifting your attention from the pain to your breathing

- using some techniques from mindfulness, like mindful stretching or meditation

- finding the best type of support and help

Stories from others with pain may be a helpful guide. Visit the websites suggested in this Footstep and discover more from other people with pain.

Difficulties with acceptance and how to overcome them

There are all sorts of reasons that you might struggle with acceptance. It takes more time than we think. It requires patience and persistence and it can be an up-and-down journey. These are some of the struggles that people with pain have shared:

- Family or friends may stay focused on finding a cure or way to fix the pain. They may not know much about persistent pain. Sharing this Footstep and others in this book may help.

- Feelings take over when you are in pain. You can easily get anxious or become angry quickly. This gets in the way of thinking about things in a balanced way. The feelings may stop you making sensible or better choices at that moment. Explore Footstep 6 on moods.

- Your mind can overreact, often with unhelpful thoughts. It is easy to jump to conclusions or think the worst and predict that things will go very wrong.

- It's hard to see any other solution or options and difficult at times to think of other ways of doing things, like changing to flexible, helpful routines.

- Lots of life's stresses can make problem-solving difficult, especially when you are distracted by pain.

Can you spot any of these struggles in yourself? Nearly everyone has similar struggles and this is partly because pain stresses both body and mind. By moving towards acceptance, and learning new self-management skills, you will find these struggles start to shrink. You will become much more confident about living well with your pain.

Shahda shares her acceptance with kindness towards herself

I know in my own life journey, coping with pain at such a young age, and that pain continuing to this day, has been tremendously challenging. I fought against it, I pushed through it but the real healing happened when I learnt acceptance and compassion towards myself. That is when everything changed. I learnt to live with the pain and the pain doesn't rage as it used to . . . I feel blessed to have the life I do.

My Footstep action plan

These are some questions to ask yourself now that you've explored more about acceptance:

* Is there one thing that I can do now to help myself with acceptance?

* What would I like to focus on next?

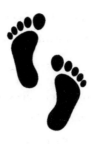

Footstep 3:

Pacing every day for better times

Everybody with persistent pain agrees that pacing is a really, really important and useful skill to learn. They say not knowing how to pace yourself means your day or activity is controlled by pain. Pacing or balancing activities help turn it the other way around.

So what is pacing?

Pacing is taking a break before pain, tiredness or exhaustion force you to stop your activities or task.

Stef's story

I was never any good at pacing even before I had neck pain. I always pushed myself harder or longer to get things done. My early life was difficult, my parents were very critical, had money problems and I had to earn money myself during my teens. This probably made me drive myself harder and it was tough to change my way of doing things. I was very dominated by the pain. I had to get back to work and so get fit quickly. I would do far too much at home or at the gym. When I got back to work I did loads of overtime to make up for the money lost when out of work. My pain took me over again. I would be off work, fed up and stuck at home often in bed or on the sofa all day.

Slowly I learnt with practice and trial and error to use pacing. It made a real difference. I found out I was using too much effort for too long. I learnt to balance my breaks and activity or work better. It was difficult as just when I felt good doing something I had to take a break. I then learnt to use breathing to slow me down and relax better. I am much more reliable now, less of a perfectionist and the family are pleased too.

Stef's story is not unusual. Many people feel their pain often controls their daily activities. They use pain to guide them so, on a 'good' day with less pain, they throw themselves into things to get as much done as possible. Then pain and tiredness increases and forces them to stop, like Stef. It is like driving as far as possible without a fuel stop on a 'feel good' sunny day. Then you run out of fuel and the car needs to be rescued!

Often, when doing an activity, your body feels good for a while, less stiff, wants to keep going and not take a rest. This type of striving often pushes on into severe pain setbacks and forces you to rest for much longer.

This is called the '**boom-and-bust cycle**' or '**overactive and collapse trap**'. It is useful for getting important things done for a crucial deadline like moving house. But it is an unhelpful thinking pattern in managing pain every day.

Pacing helps avoid the boom-and-bust cycle. It puts you, not your pain, in charge. If you can get into the routine of pacing, you can do more things with partners, family and friends and have a fuller life.

How to pace well

It's important to realise that pacing skills take time to learn and you need to practise endless times over weeks to become confident using them. Pacing means finding the balance between what your mind wants you to do or you have to do and what is kinder for you and your body. It is planning and giving yourself regular rest breaks and time to re-store energy: in other words, *planning the route and your refuelling stops*.

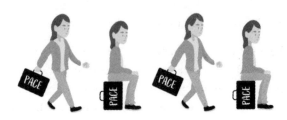

Activity - Rest - Repeat

1. Decide which activities you need to pace

Think about your daily activities and how much effort they require. If any of these activities are difficult because of your pain, or if pain increases as you do them, then they probably need to be paced.

2. Find how much effort to put into each activity without causing more pain

It can be tricky to work out what effort level is right for you. So, for example, say walking to the local store is difficult. First, find how far you can walk before your pain starts or increases.

Think about:

- What is the speed at which I can do the activity? Slow, medium or fast pace?

- How far can I walk without more pain or tiredness?

- How often do I need to take rest breaks?

Let's say you can usually walk 200 metres to a store at a medium pace and then the pain increases. To pace the activity, reduce 200 metres by half, and take a break at 100 metres. You can slow down your pace to manage energy too.

Take a break of, say, five minutes and then pace the walk, both the speed and effort, for the next 100 metres. Take a rest break again. Now you have walked into the store, 200 metres away, with little change in pain.

Use pacing for other activities – tasks around the garden or house, social events, work, etc. Discover how much you can do until the pain increases or interferes with the activity. Reduce the activity to half this amount, put in breaks and complete it. It is a truly useful habit. Others have shared that *'Pain is life-changing and daunting, so always break activities down into chunks, tackle them one by one and even if you are taking baby steps, you will still move forward.'*

Using regular breaks you can do more throughout the day, with less pain or tiredness, and you will steadily build up body stamina.

Amy's story

Amy loved dancing but stopped going to her local dance class with her friends as it made her spinal pain worse. She decided it was too much effort, too painful and tiring. This changed when she learnt the skill of pacing.

Amy realised that she didn't have to join in every dance like the others so she planned to do the easy, slower dances or every third dance and then rest. Her plans turned out well. She had fun and discovered she was less tired than she expected. She felt happier as she was doing something she enjoyed with her friends.

---

3. Be aware of how your body feels in the moment

You may find that if you are feeling tired or stiff or have more pain than usual, it helps to take a few extra breaks or give less effort to the activity. This isn't always easy as your mind may be telling you to get the job done *now* or finish the activity *today*, despite your pain. Think how to achieve a balance between what you *want* to do and what you *can* do without increasing your pain.

Experiment with the balance between effort, activity and pain and/or tiredness to find the kindest level for you.

Tools and tips to help pace well

Pacing needs practice every day and works well with goal setting (see Footstep 4). People with pain find these tips help them:

- In a break time, have a chair or bench to sit on. Do some simple stretches. Listen to some pleasant music.

- Use a timer from your kitchen or on a mobile phone to tell you when it's time to take a break.

- Add in a drink break to your activity plan. Use a timer to make the break long enough!

- Ring a friend or make a phone call as a break.

- Try the relaxation breathing ideas in Footstep 9.

Ways to deal with difficulties with pacing

You will have found out already that your mind can get in the way! It's common to fall into the '*all-or-nothing thinking*' trap. You set off on a task and think, 'I've started, so I'll finish it now'. It is hard to accept that some things can be finished later. Or, like Amy and dancing, you may stop doing something you enjoy altogether as you can't do it as you used to. This way of thinking is very common. It is a block to pacing well and pushes you into pain setbacks.

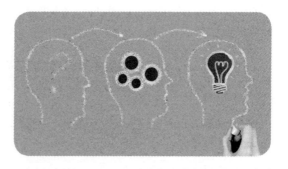

Pacing needs *balanced thinking* and these ideas may help:

- Notice unhelpful thoughts like 'must' or 'should' and replace with *'could'*. For example, instead of thinking 'I must get it all done today', try thinking 'I could choose to pace this and do it in stages over two or more days'. Experiment and see what actually gets done without more pain.

- Let go of the idea that all the jobs get done today. It is not giving in, *except* to pain!

- Prioritise – tell yourself some things can be done later, tomorrow or next week.

- Tell the people around you that you are practising pacing – maybe share this Footstep. Ask for their support to help you pace well.

- Check the effort levels of the activity. This skill of matching effort and activity helps make certain the balance is right for the situation or plan. A low effort level means things may not get done, may take ages and frustration may move in with the lack of progress. But too much effort and you crash out with a setback.

So treat it like checking the temperature in an oven. Too little heat and the dish is undercooked; too much heat and the dish burns. An effort scale guides the balance of your activity to prevent a pacing disaster. *(See Footstep 4: Set goals, action plans and rewards, and Footstep 5: Getting fit and staying active.)*

Effort Scale For Pacing Activities and Goals

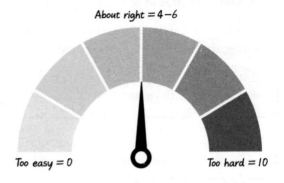

Rate your effort level for an activity on the scale below

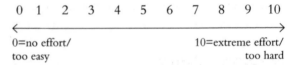

Figure 1. Effort scale

Give an effort level to the activities you pace. If your score is between 4 and 6 then this is the balanced range of effort to succeed.

If effort level on scale is:

<u>3 or less</u>   spend more time on the activity *and/<u>or</u>* do it with more speed or effort

<u>8 or more</u>   reduce it with more breaks *and/or* shorter time for activity

---

Balancing the body and mind together on activities helps do what *you* want to do. This will help you to control your pain and life with more success and less stress and to move on in your life journey.

Give pacing a go – start with a pacing plan and reward yourself for achieving a helpful habit for life.

My Footstep action plan

ABC questions to pace activities:

A. What **A**ctivities can I pace today or this week?

B. How long before I take a **B**reak/s? _____ minutes

C. **C**heck the effort level on the scale.

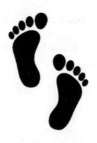

Footstep 4:

Set goals, action plans and rewards

This Footstep is about creating simple step-by-step action plans to achieve your goals. This skill helps you to get on with life and discover kinder ways to live well.

Learning to self-manage your pain is a journey and it's never a good idea to set out on a journey without a map. People with pain find that making goals, and planning how to achieve them, helps them stay on course and make progress.

What do we mean by goal setting?

Goal setting is about focusing on the things in your life that you want to change. You can think about any area of your life, such as:

- Building a fit body and mind

- Fun/enjoyable activities: hobbies, sports, events or celebrations

- Relaxation to reduce stress, unwind the body and mind

- Your role in life or work, doing jobs around the home or family time

Start with fairly easy goals such as:

- Read a chosen book within the next month

- Pot plants in the greenhouse by the end of May

- Learn some relaxing yoga or stretches in the next six weeks

- Meet friends and go to the Wednesday football match

- Swim and relax in the sauna every week

- Walk for thirty minutes daily for the next month

Then use your experience to move on to more challenging goals. Try to make sure your goals are SMART:

S = **Specific:** they specify clearly what you want to achieve.

M = **Meaningful:** they really matter to you.

A = **Achievable:** they require some effort but are not too difficult.

R = **Realistic:** they can be achieved alongside your other roles and commitments. For example, setting a relaxation goal mid-afternoon may not work if children are due home from school.

T = **Time-based:** they can be achieved within a certain amount of time – ideally within a few weeks or a couple of months.

Planning your steps to achieve your goals

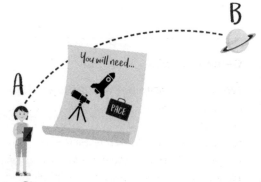

Action Planning

If your goal is the end destination, you need to work out how you are going to get there. This is what action planning is about.

So for example, Pete Moore's goal was to *'get fit enough to walk two kilometres around the local paths by the end of two months'*. He knew that he would have to work up to achieving it, so he created an action plan with these questions:

- **WHAT will help me achieve my goal?** Stretches and some walking exercise to build my fitness

- **HOW much do I need to do?** Around thirty minutes every day

- **WHEN will I do it?** Monday–Saturday

- **HOW OFTEN?** Split over two sessions, in the morning and late afternoon

---

Getting the effort level right

Pete wanted to make sure that he wasn't asking too much of himself, so he thought about how much effort was needed for his action plan. He used the effort scale of 0–10 where 0 is too easy/ no effort and 10 is too hard/totally exhausting. He decided that to go ahead he needed an effort score of 5–7. If the score was above 7, then he could set himself up for disappointment.

Pete rated his action plan with an effort level of 8, so a bit too high!!

Effort Scale For Pacing Activities and Goals

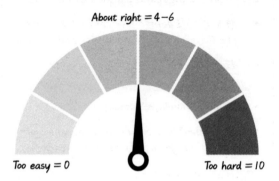

What kind of things could Pete change to adjust his effort level?

He could do a number of things, such as:

1. Reduce the:

- number of days that he did his stretches and exercises

- amount of time he spent doing his stretches and exercises

2. Add a reward for doing the plan the first three times

3. Share his plan with other people and get their support

Pete made changes and planned this instead:

- **What am I doing?** *Five arm and leg stretches plus five minutes' walking exercise to build fitness*

- **How much?** *For twenty minutes with one break*

- **When?** *Monday–Saturday*

- **How often?** *Split over two sessions, in the morning and late afternoon for the next seven days*

The effort level for Pete's new plan was 6, so he was good to go!

Remember how easy it is to make a plan that ends with too much effort, especially if your pain levels are low at the time. The effort scale (0–10 score) helps check you are not striving too hard. The kinder effort level is between 5 and 7.

Tips for good goals and action plans

- Write down goals that will make you feel good. If the goal makes you cringe, wince or feel worried, then cross it out. Positive feelings, rewards and support are all crucial for success.

- Have goals you can achieve, even on difficult days with pain.

- Remember that making and completing an action plan is a success in itself. Every time you do something on your action plan you move closer to your goal.

- Use positive coping talk like, '*I enjoy the planning and I know I can do the goal if I take each step steadily, with breaks. I like what Pete suggests.*'

- Watch out for unhelpful thinking like, '*I can't do this*' or put-downs like, '*it failed last time so it will this time*' or, '*I am not good at this stuff*'.

- Imagine a best friend struggling with his/her action plan. Try to make some suggestions to him/her. Then share these with yourself to guide you.

- Share your goal and action plan with others. Ask for support and listen to their ideas to help you succeed.

- Imagine that you reached your goal/s. What would you say to yourself and other people? What reward would you give yourself for all your effort?

True stories of goal success!

Tosh had some bad news at the pain service. Major side effects meant his planned treatment would not be possible. His GP helped him to see he needed to be fitter. This pushed him to get his fitness on track. He decided to learn to road cycle again despite his back pain. His goal was to 'ride five kilometres on the local cycle path within the next eight weeks'. He did an action plan for the first two weeks and saw he had an effort level of 9/10. He talked this through with Sam, his partner, and made changes to it.

Tosh steadily progressed towards his eight-week goal despite some ups and downs and a puncture on his road bike. In weeks three and four he actually rode up the road. He felt excited, kept on with gym cycling and slowly increased his road cycle time. By week five, he had reached the cycle path a mile from his house. His confidence grew, he was upbeat and he reminded himself not to over pace again. He felt wiser now, as he'd done that before!

One year later . . . Tosh cycled 100 kilometres, raising money for a cancer charity, and had found part-time work he enjoyed. His reward – a new fishing rod!

Rewarding yourself

Rewards can help you to make positive progress towards your goals. They can increase your drive

Tosh's first action plan		Tosh's second action plan	
What am I doing?	Cycling to Bishopton	**What am I doing?**	Cycling on a static bike at the gym
How much?	2 kilometres away	**How much?**	1 kilometre on low setting
When?	10 a.m.	**When?**	10.30 at the gym
How often?	Monday, Thursday and Sunday	**How often?**	Tuesday, Thursday, Sunday
Effort level	9/10	**Effort level**	5/10
'I'll fail with this plan' — CANCEL IT		*'Much better, much easier'* — SPOT ON	

to carry out new activities or make changes in your routine. People with pain find that giving themselves regular, kind and pleasurable rewards really motivates them to become a 'can do it' person.

Explore Bob's story of change after his struggle for twenty years with back pain and see what you learn from his experience:

Bob's story

I was always striving to be fitter and to stop walking with my crutches. I hated them and myself for being quite so weak. Then I found that I could do static walking at the gym. I found a buddy, Samjee, who liked walking outdoors too and we planned walks together. We found the canal was a sensible route to start on and we had regular stops to enjoy the views and wildlife. Over weeks we built it up and rewarded ourselves with a café stop at the end of the walk. We kept a record with photos on our mobile phones of how far we had walked since we started. This shifted my 'cannot do this' thinking. I was keener and more strong-minded to walk most days.

We kept up the regular walks and it's hard to believe that over the next year I lost weight —

> *4 stone. I found myself a different, stronger and fitter person. Giving myself rewards worked well – the best one was booking my first holiday overseas with my wife, Pam!*

Reward tips

Make the reward personal to you, like Bob did, as something that is a reward for one person may not be rewarding for another.

Little or big rewards are fine. You can choose to use them for each action plan as well as the final goal. Experiment and do only what works to build your motivation and confidence.

Make rewards interesting by using smell, colour, sound, taste and touch to satisfy your different senses. You could watch a 'feel good' movie with great music and have a fruity smoothie drink. This helps retrain the brain to focus on other things than your pain and to make the changes you want.

More examples are:

- A hot shower with nice perfumed shower gel listening to your favourite music

- Read your favourite hobby magazine for a set time

- Meet friends for chat and drink in a nice café or place

It helps to give your rewards a pleasure level, 0 = no pleasure and 10 = extremely pleasurable. Pleasure levels of 6 or more help activities or tasks succeed and tell you what type of rewards work well for you.

My action plan

Goal setting is a key skill and needs plans of action to chart the journey and measure progress.

Explore the Goal Ladder in Appendix 1 for more ideas.

My goal is .... (SMART)

My first two steps on my action plans are ....

....

....

What are my effort levels?

What are my rewards for progress?

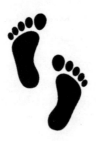

Footstep 5:

Getting fit and staying active

An enjoyable, rewarding and regular activity plan builds confidence to do things and lessens the struggles with pain. People with pain say being more active and building fitness helps them even if it was *not* really part of their life before pain arrived. This Footstep guides you to build up your activities and fitness steadily and works well with Footstep 3: Pacing and Footstep 4: Set goals, action plans and rewards.

Why get fit?

Pete Moore shares what he discovered about being fitter:

'Getting fitter and more active played a major factor in reducing my pain. At the start I was one of those people who thought that exercise equalled more pain. It did in

the early days, as I tried too hard to do too much, too soon and too fast — I over paced it!

'*Many people with pain like me stop keeping active because when we move it hurts, then our muscles become weak and unsteady and our joints get what I call "rusty".*

'*It's true that when we start stretching and exercising pain levels can increase, but they soon drop off. Look at it this way: if a door has not been opened for some time, the hinges may creak a bit. When we move the door backwards and forwards a few times . . . it stops creaking. It's the same with our joints and body.*

'*For me getting fitter means not having to take pain medication. I haven't done so for the past few years. Stretching and exercising are my daily doses of medicine. The only side effects are **less** pain and feeling good about myself!!*

'*The key to getting fitter is to explore some ideas, get started and keep it going every day.*'

How can I get fitter and more active?

Your plan needs to contain:

1. Stretching to loosen tight muscles, ligaments and joints and increase your flexibility. Stretching prepares the body for movement and activity and helps improve posture.

2. Strengthening exercises to build stronger muscles and joints so that you can stand, walk and play for longer. These will help you to get out of chairs and use stairs and slopes more easily. Your balance will improve and this reduces the chances of falls and pain setbacks.

3. Stamina activities to help you to do things for longer without more pain or tiredness. These help you to enjoy a range of day-to-day activities, join in with family and friends and have less fear of more pain.

The tricky bit is deciding what to do, how to do it, how much time and effort to put in and who can help. It's a good idea to set goals and make some action plans to succeed. Check Footstep 4: Set goals, action plans and rewards to guide you and do not forget to pace these goals so use Footstep 3: Pacing to help.

Some ideas from Pete Moore to guide your plans:

1. Choose something easy and fun to do, like

- A gentle walk in a favourite place – pace the time and length

- Stretching and listening to your favourite radio programme

- Gentle yoga or Pilates, guided by a DVD, website or app (see resources)

- Volunteering in a museum, public garden or library

- Dancing to enjoyable music at home

- Planting out bedding plants in tubs or in the garden

2. Explore fitness and activity choices where you live. It can be a fitness group – and anything that involves moving and stretching, like a pottery class or a singing group, is fine.

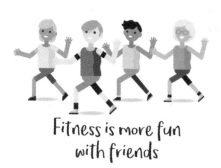

Fitness is more fun
with friends

3. Do some activities with other people. This will boost or motivate you to keep up your activity levels, find new ways to be active and build up your own 'support team'.

Mick's story

Mick struggled to get fit and reduce weight so felt fed up. He avoided his local pool as sometimes it was too hot and made him very tired and sweaty. A friend, Frank, told him about an adult swim and fitness group for people with health problems, saying, 'I am going next week, come with me, if you like.' Mick swallowed hard and felt nervous and then plucked up courage: 'I'll give it a go.' At the pool, Mick and Frank discovered that other people swimming had similar pain problems. He felt encouraged so swam two lengths of the pool and decided to go again the next week.

---

4. Keeping motivated. This can be a tough one. If the activity you choose is too much effort, *do something else*. Of course, do not start with something that requires an effort level of 9 where 10 means too hard, totally exhausting!! Do something with an effort level of 4 to 6 and build up fitness steadily. Give yourself regular *rewards* for your successes. Share them with other people so that they notice your progress and support you.

How to make progress

1. Set one or two goals and make a plan to achieve them

2. Use the effort scale idea in Footstep 4: Setting goals, action plan and rewards to guide you to a fair balance of activity and fitness and rest breaks. This will stop you pushing into more pain.

Effort Scale For Pacing Activities and Goals

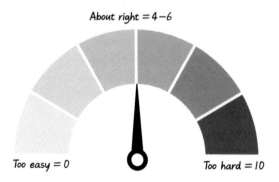

About right = 4–6

Too easy = 0

Too hard = 10

3. If the effort level needed is more above 7 or 8 out of 10, look at ways to reduce the effort to a 4–6 level when working on your fitness.

4. Be ready and organised. Have the right kit ready, like comfortable footwear or swimwear + towel. It helps you think 'I can just go now and do it . . . ' and you are less likely to get sidetracked from your plan.

5. Watch for any 'put down' and 'can't do' or 'what if' thinking as it can sabotage your efforts. Write down unhelpful thoughts, or share them with someone who supports you, and then let them go.

Mick's progress

Mick went to the pool next time with Frank. He worked out his effort level of 6/10 and baseline swimming distance and swam four lengths in forty minutes. He did one length at a time with a five-minute break. He even walked a pool length to help his muscles to climb out of the pool more easily. He expected more pain again as his muscles had ached after the first swim. He did ache again, of course, but he was not hot or sweaty and noticed his swimming was easier. He felt less grumpy and tired and told Frank that he had enjoyed it.

Dealing with difficulties

Many people still use their pain as a guide as to when to start and stop an activity. This is the pain managing you – it's not *you managing pain*!!

The main thing to remember is that when you begin to stretch and exercise, it is normal for pain levels to increase. The good news is, these pains soon go away *if you grade your activities*. Grading means gently increasing the amount of time you spend doing your stretches, exercises or fitness plan. For example:

Stretching: *(Keep your effort level at 5/6 for the activity)*

Day one: hold a stretch for 5 seconds and do three repeats

Day two: hold a stretch for 6 seconds and do three repeats

Day three: hold a stretch for 7 seconds . . . and so on

Over the next few days slowly build up the repeats and time on stretching.

Exercise: *For walking find the distance you can do before your pain starts to increase. If this distance is 100 metres, reduce it by half. This 50 metres distance is your baseline and your start point to build fitness by walking.*

Day one: walk for 50 metres, stop for a break of two to five minutes. Walk 50 metres more so that you have walked 100 metres without lots more pain.

Keep up for a week walking 100 metres (still with rests) and graded stretching every day. Slowly your baseline increases over the weeks and months.

Remember that you are in charge of the fitness plan and if you experience much more pain, you may have done too much, too quickly. You may need to tweak your baseline and check out your effort level, the speed and the length of the activity. Use relaxation breathing for some minutes after graded stretching and help the muscles relax and unwind. Motivate yourself with rewards often.

Finally, getting fit and staying active despite pain helps the brain to turn down your pain system sensitivity. Explore more about the pain and brain in Footstep 2. Getting fitter helps your brain to process pain messages in more helpful ways and lessen your pain and stress. Best of all you become more independent and more confident.

More useful resources

Find a Chartered Physiotherapist or fitness trainer/ coach if you are struggling. Check if they have specific experience in working with people with pain. They can guide your stretch programme and help you to improve balance and posture, and strengthen unfit muscles and joints. http://www.csp.org.uk/ your-health/find-physio/find-physiotherapist

Handy tip: Check NHS Choices Fitness Studio for exercise videos and learn yoga, tai chi and Pilates at your own pace at home. It's open 24 hours a day,

365 days of the year and is free. http://www.nhs.uk/conditions/nhs-fitness-studio

My action plan

Try these questions:

1. What enjoyable fitness activity can I start now?

2. Do I want to become fitter on my own or along with people?

3. What's my baseline for walking or any other activity?

4. How do I progress my baseline?

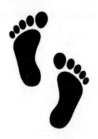

Footstep 6:

Managing moods

It is normal to struggle with moods when you have persistent pain. Emotions or moods linked to pain are difficult to manage and can take over day-to-day life. People with pain find that positive management of their mood changes makes a valuable difference to their pain and their lives.

What do we mean by 'managing moods'?

We all go through periods of 'moodiness' when we feel irritable, sad, frustrated or worried. Although the feelings are not very pleasant at the time, they do tend to pass, and soon we feel happier or more content.

People with pain often find they feel:

- Angry and frustrated

- Fearful and worried

- Low and unmotivated

If you have these feelings then you probably find that they get in the way of your day-to-day life and can be overwhelming at times. It is common to think that there is nothing you can do as they just 'take over' and go on for a long time. This is because these mood changes come from the struggle of living with pain. This is *not your fault.* It is more about how our human mind works when it is stressed with pain, we feel unwell or deal with difficult life events. The mind is trying to make sense of everything that is happening and cope with it all.

The good news is that you can do things to manage your moods better. Discover more in this Footstep.

Why is this important?

Many people with pain find that the more knowledge and ways they have to cope with moods, the better their life and confidence gets.

Denise's story

Denise e-mailed this post to Ask Pete www.pain-toolkit.org.uk

'I've tried yoga, acupuncture, chiropractors, Pilates, massage therapy, hot/cold treatments and nothing seems to make the pain go away. Last week, my dad, who is a physiotherapist, thought that my pain might not be physical any more and might be psychological. I get really frustrated as whatever I do, the pain is still there. My friends have noticed I am much more irritable and tearful.

I'm just not sure what to do any more. I had big dreams and plans for myself. Things look much bleaker and I just want to feel good about myself and life again. I don't know how or if it's even possible any more.

Please, let me know what you think and if you have any advice or suggestions, I'm open to trying anything.'

Pete shared the Pain and Living-my-life-well circles (see the Introduction) and acceptance ideas with Denise to help her understand why she struggled with moods. This helped her to step back and see how her mood, thoughts and pain were all connected. She saw how her mind shifted into negative thinking 'I can't do or can't be' patterns about herself which reduced her motivation and made her frustrated and down.

The Living-my-life-well circle gave her hope to try new ways to track and deal with unhelpful moods and thoughts. This helped her angry or 'grumpy' moods lessen. She found she was making progress and started on new plans for work and doing things with friends.

Like Denise, you may find that your thoughts start being negative or follow frustrating patterns. You may have thoughts like, 'I'm useless now', 'I'll never do that again', 'Things are not going to work out' and 'No-one seems to understand me now or want to help'. It is like a tape recording in your head, which no one else hears. Realistic positive changes can come from learning to deal with these unhelpful thoughts. Look at the tools and techniques below and decide how you can put them into practice and make yourself an action plan.

Ways to manage moods better?

Practise kindness and compassion

Being kind and compassionate to yourself is one of the best things that you can do. It's very easy to be self-critical and beat yourself up for not being perfect or not getting the job done. But the more you do this, the more likely it is that negative and unkind thoughts will emerge. This pushes your pain networks into stress mode, they become more sensitive and so pain and distress increase.

So trying to be a 100 per cent person all the time can be unhelpful. Instead, ask yourself, *'What is kind and caring for me, my body or mind right now?'* Experiment and do things that lessen the stress or pressure. This will help your body's opioids – the pain-reducing chemicals – to work better and soothe some of the pain and upset in your mind. This in turn can reduce some of the adrenaline levels that increase stressful pressure and symptoms.

Remember that it is *'not your fault'* that the pain refuses to go away. So how can you help lessen the stress or pressure? Below are nine ways to work with moods which other people found helpful. Discover which ones work for you and then use them often.

Some mood management tools and tips

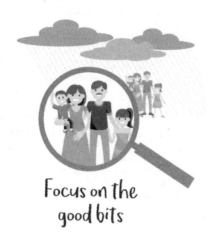

Focus on the
good bits

1. Notice negative unhelpful thoughts that affect your mood as soon as you can. They are powerful and believable because they creep in without you noticing them, but if you get into the habit of spotting them quickly you can use different methods to balance or soothe them.

2. Practise balanced thinking. Write down some of your negative thoughts and then imagine what a best friend would say if they knew you were thinking them. Make a note of this and use it when they pop back into your mind. You will also see that these negative thoughts are not always 100 per cent true and believable.

3. Do things that unwind and soothe your mind, like walking the dog, listening to music, doodling, breathing calmly or doing craft activities, even knitting . . . anything that is calming.

4. Build a list of positive things you have done that day or week. This will show you that you are coping or managing life, despite the pain. This positive facts diary helps deal with 'can't do this' thinking. You'll find that you are doing positive things. It is just that your mind gets too distracted and focused on negative thinking at times. Here is Mario's example of a positive fact diary.

Mario's positive fact sheet

It is a struggle to cope with the leg pains. These things put me back in control again.

Monday: The stretches all through the day made me more flexible.

Wednesday: I am coping with work 40 per cent better than three months ago.

Saturday: Two setbacks in three weeks were just minor ones, still did the shopping with Rosa!

Sunday: More rewards for my effort and progress – 'booked to see the new film at cinema'.

I need to remember how far I have come, my confidence is better; even Rosa, my wife, says so.

Plan on Monday: Speak with the manager at work to change my hours.

KEY TIP: Use your mobile phone to take photos of your positive moments – a quick and easy way to collect facts and have a visible record!

5. Practise being kind to yourself. For instance: check you are balancing activities and effort; work towards fun goals in paced steps; do something enjoyable, like have a meal out with a friend.

6. Learn from others with similar pain issues. Find out what other people do to deal with negative thinking and moods through local support groups or useful websites (check the Resources section at the end of this book).

7. Get into helpful habits. Find what made a really useful change for you last week and then use it again this week.

8. Discover other ways to tackle moods with negative thinking. Self-help resources to manage moods can be found in most local libraries or you can explore the websites suggested at the end of this book.

9. Share your plans with people you trust and get their support. Remember that you are not alone. We all need support and encouragement from other people, so do not feel bad about asking friends and family to help you.

Specific moods and how to deal with them

Anger

Pain research has found that dealing with anger is really important. When people have a sense of unfairness about their pain and its impact on their life, they tend to struggle more with pain itself.

A lot of unfair things may have happened in your journey with pain. Unhelpful or unkind things may have been said to you or you may have missed out on opportunities because of it. This can add to feelings of anger.

Here are some ideas to help you work through anger – find out what works better for you:

- Share your feelings with someone you trust to gain a more balanced way of viewing the unfairness or injustice that causes difficulties for you.

- Channel your anger in a positive direction. Some people use their anger and its energy to motivate themselves to address an issue in a positive way.

> *For example, Mario set up 'SMILE', a supportive self-management group for people with pain. He had learnt the skills to be confident and less angry and wanted to support others to make changes to cope better with pain. 'Five years was too long before I discovered how to self-manage well.'*

*   Deal with the adrenaline release that comes with anger. A method that many people have found incredibly useful is OTSAR breathing (Appendix 2). This key breathing technique helps you to unwind and calms the mind and body in a few minutes.

*   When anger starts, ask yourself, '*Is it really worth it?*'. Take a break to calm and wind down to reassess the issue and situation.

Anxiety

Anxiety is a mood that winds up the sensitivity of the pain systems. Anxiety and worry affect the way you think about yourself, other people, the future and your pain. You find you tend to:

- Over-estimate the fearful problem or threat

- Under-estimate your ability to cope or make yourself safe

- Ignore the things that reduce or limit the danger or threat.

Four suggestions that people with pain have found helped lessen anxiety:

1. Reduce caffeine from all sources of drink and food. Jackie's's experience shows that this can make a big difference to how your body feels.

Jackie's story

Jackie realised that she drank twenty cups of coffee a day to perk herself up as she did not sleep well. So she cut down the cups of coffee over a fortnight and found that many of her sensations, like chest thumping, stopped. Her fitness improved too, so her legs felt less 'wobbly' and she became less scared of falling down the stairs. Six weeks later she found herself confidently climbing flights of steps in a football stadium, by pacing it.

---

2. Use relaxation skills, especially belly breathing and OTSAR (APPENDIX 2).

3. Watch out for negative anxious thinking and try some of the tools and tips suggested earlier.

4. Do experiments and see if your fears or worries about the pain or its effects come true 100 per cent of the time. For example, if you are scared that the pain will worsen when you do some new or more stretches, then experiment. Try out one or two more or new stretches, using breathing to guide the movements. Then see what actually happens. The pain is very likely to be unchanged. Continue to repeat again the same stretches and increase the repetitions by one or two. Slowly build up the time and amount of stretching. Discover what actually happens to your pain levels. Check Footsteps 3–5 to guide you too.

5. To explore more about anxiety or anger moods follow the links at end of the book.

Loss and sadness

Pain has a big impact and many people say that they feel a sense of loss and sadness because of how pain has affected their life. Often these losses are not recognised by others, so pain leads to being more lost and isolated. This type of grief is normal. Recognising it, and sharing your feelings with people you trust, can make things easier. It takes time to adjust to these losses and find new ways to be confident and build goals. There is a lot you can do for yourself, or, like Denise, you might need some help.

Denise's story

Denise found it hard to cope with the feelings of loss that came with living with pain. She was no longer fit and healthy. She missed doing things with her friends. She couldn't go to college so she felt she had lost her future. It was only through talking with a counsellor that she was able to view her situation more positively and make some plans for her future.

Seeking help

If you find you are really struggling with low or anxious moods and negative thinking, then see your doctor or local healthcare service for help. They can help and work out with you what kind of talking therapy or other treatments might bene-fit you. Sometimes pain, or difficult or traumatic events from the past, can make moods more intense, unpredictable and difficult to deal with and extra help can make a real difference.

My Action Plan

These are some questions to guide your action plan, suggested by people with pain (like Mario, Jackie and Denise). Discover what works well for you and explore the useful resources at the end of this book.

1. What moods shall I work on now? If I feel stuck, what would a best friend suggest?

2. When shall I work on my mood? Today, this week?

3. What will I try to help me have better moods?

4. How can I reward myself for my actions?

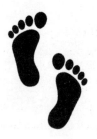

Footstep 7:

Sleep well more often

Most people with pain find their sleep is disrupted regularly and they need help to sleep better and well. They find the struggle to sleep, combined with their reactions to sleeping badly, actually makes it all much worse!

You may have tried all sorts of ways to improve your sleep and even think there is little now you can do. New research on sleep and pain management has found that sleeping well is possible and needs a different approach and maybe new skills.

What causes sleep problems?

People with pain find these are the six most common triggers or stresses:

1. Pain itself

It's hard to get off to sleep when you feel pain. It is quiet and there are no other distractions. Pain is the main focus of your mind. You notice it more so you have more body tension and worries. The more you struggle with sleep and pain, the harder it is to fall asleep. It is a vicious circle like in Pat's story below.

2. Bedroom comfort

Perhaps the only place where pain is less is in a lying position in bed or on a sofa. However, this can lead to stiffness and tightness in muscles and joints. This added pain can stop restful sleep. Then the bed can feel too hard or too soft. Noise from outside or inside the bedroom can affect sleep, like snoring from other people. Frustration sets in with more pain and less sleep – another unhelpful circle.

3. Mood changes

If you are anxious or low, then you may have troubling or worrying thoughts. These take over your mind and, along with pain, creating more tension in your body, making it even harder to fall and stay asleep.

4. Lack of routine and daytime inactivity

Regular routines can be tricky when you have pain. A bad day with pain puts plans and activities out of routine and then you try to catch up on a 'good day'. Irregular routines confuse the body and mind so they no longer *know* when to be active or to rest.

5. Unhelpful thinking about poor sleep

Sometimes you and your worry about how a lack of sleep will affect you the next day. Your mind goes over things and even makes worrying predictions. The body gets more tense and painful, adrenaline levels rise, your heart may race and you get restless and stay awake. Then at last you fall asleep and wake up tired. Another unhelpful circle!

6. Side effects of medicines

Medicines for pain and mood can interfere with sleep patterns in many ways. They can make you drowsy in the day. This can lead to going to sleep much later or earlier than your usual sleep time. Slowly the day and night pattern of activity of the body and mind changes.

Pat's sleepless story

Pat was exhausted, fed up as his back pain meant he had not had a full night's sleep for weeks. Josie, his wife, snored, so he was often woken up. He spent some nights in bed or on the sofa. Rows with Josie did not help. She was tired and upset too. He tried, on better days, to do more around the house to help Josie but then got more pain. Being grumpy and worried just added to his tiredness and 'bad sleep'.

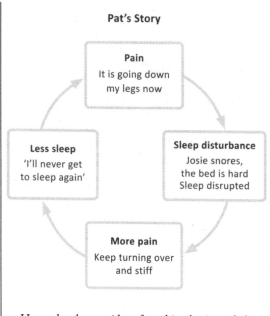

Pat's Story

Pain
It is going down
my legs now

Sleep disturbance
Josie snores,
the bed is hard
Sleep disrupted

More pain
Keep turning over
and stiff

Less sleep
'I'll never get
to sleep again'

He explored some ideas from his physio and the booklets at the end of this book. He changed some of his routine using the ideas below.

How to sleep well despite pain

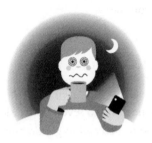

To sleep well, help your body recharge, be alert, focused and have happier moods, there are two helpful things you can do:

- Take control of activities and keep to routines

- Be more accepting of those things that you can't control and *lessen this stress*

This balance leads to better sleep and a sense of wellness.

Sleeping well is about what you do at night *and* in the day, so take control in these four areas:

1. Daily routines

2. Activity levels

3. Food and drink choices

4. Bedtime routines

1. Your daily routines

Most adults need seven to eight hours' sleep; older people only need six to seven hours' sleep. A regular time to go to bed and to get up helps the mind's waking and sleep centres run a balanced on-and-off system. These centres can get very confused by changes in routine, like jet lag from plane travel or changing night shift work.

A regular routine helps the body and mind know when it is time to relax and sleep or to be alert. Other activities need regular times, like when you:

•   Get up from sleep and settle to sleep

•   Eat and drink

•   Are active

So find your better daily routine, and stick with it whatever happens for several weeks, even in setbacks.

Eddie's story

Eddie, an ex-postman, found that it worked well to start his day at 5 a.m. He did some gentle stretches under a warm shower and walked the dog. He saw his daughter over breakfast and helped his wife, Tracy, before she left for work. After they left, he did fifteen-minutes' breathing relaxation to pace his morning before going to his part-time job. He'd accepted now the odd bad night's sleep. Tracy helped him to stick better to morning and night routines, including eating by 7 p.m. and having decaffeinated drinks at night.

Eddie no longer had a two-hour afternoon nap. Instead he stayed awake by doing more stretches, talking with Tracy and doing mindfulness practice. After three months, he was sleeping around seven hours until 5.30 a.m. with an odd wakeful night. He woke with more energy, was more cheerful when Tracy came back from work. He even danced her around the kitchen and they laughed more.

---

2. Your activity levels

Pain can affect your confidence to do any kind of

physical activity. Too little activity can affect your ability to sleep well. Small steady changes in activity through the day can make a difference, so experiment and use Footstep 5: Getting fit and staying active to guide you. Avoid energetic exercise shortly before sleep. Try gentle stretches to reduce painful stiffness instead.

3. Look at your food and drink routines

Caffeinated foods and drinks like tea, coffee, energy drinks, cola and chocolate activate the body and mind. Use them less or stop them late in the day or evening. Nicotine stimulates the body too. People who smoke in the evening often find it is hard to fall asleep and stay asleep. Think about the time of day that you eat, and the type and amount of foods that you eat. Eating a big meal before sleep time will fire your digestive system into action and your body will struggle to relax and sleep well. Lots to drink before bed may mean you wake up needing the toilet!

4. Your bedtime routine

Four practical things to do before sleep time:

a. Follow the same 'wind-down' activities every evening, like having a relaxing bath, listening to soothing music, doing some relaxation practice, reading an enjoyable magazine. Do not look at your smartphone or tablet. The screen light they emit can trick your body/mind into thinking that it is daytime, making you stay awake longer.

b. Only go to your bedroom when it is time for sleep. Do not watch television, go on the internet or do paperwork in bed. This confuses your body as these activities make you more alert. Your body and mind need to realise that your bedroom is a place for sleep.

c. Make sure your bedroom is dark, quiet and at a comfortable temperature. Block early-morning light out with thick curtains or blinds. Close windows or wear earplugs to block out noise.

d. If you don't fall asleep within fifteen to twenty minutes, then get out of bed, go into another room and do a quiet wind-down activity. Have one ready, like a jigsaw puzzle. This helpful habit helps to stop the worry about sleep. Get back into bed when you feel tired. Repeat again if you don't go to sleep.

Some skills and tools to help you sleep well

Relaxation skills help to soothe your mind and body, so use them every bedtime. They can be very powerful because they help you to *stop struggling, bring acceptance and reduce the frustration of being awake.* View things in a different way like: *I am allowing my body to rest in bed and I accept that I am just awake at this moment. There is nothing more that I can, or need to do.*

Breathing tip to help you to relax and soothe the body:

• Breath in, breath out, count 1

• Breath in, breath out, count 2

If you get to ten, start again at one and so on . . . until you fall asleep.

> *When Eddie is awake at night he thinks, 'Being awake is just fine, my body is resting in the best place.' If tension creeps up, he uses breathing skills to help him relax. Sometimes he uses the OTSAR relaxation (in Appendix 2) if feeling angry or upset.*

More on sleeping well

People wonder about using medication to help with sleep. Explore this with your doctor, as sleeping tablets are not used long-term in any pain or health problems. They are sometimes used for very short periods where the person has a clear action plan of goals they wish to achieve and are actively learning to live well with pain. Nearly all people with pain avoid these medications as they often make their days a drowsy, sleepy time, which is not their goal! If you are on medication for sleep and feel confident about trying to reduce it, *do not suddenly stop*. This 'all or nothing' action can cause a lot of distress in the body. It is kinder to reduce your medication in a steady, planned way. Your GP or specialist pain team or nurse can help support your plans.

You may have tried the 'sleep well' tips and skills suggested here over many weeks and still struggle with sleep problems. If so, explore the resources. Talking therapies called Cognitive Behavioural Therapy (CBT) or Acceptance and Commitment Therapy (ACT) can help by working through traumatic or anxious times to help guide ways to manage sleep and learn mindfulness approaches.

If you have issues of obesity, snoring or poor sleep then explore this with your doctor or clinical team. A condition called sleep apnoea could be the cause and is treatable. Explore more on the NHS Choices website.

My action plan

My plan for sleeping well includes.........................

Some hints – check:

1. The bedroom is dark, quiet, right temperature; no screen time

2. No stimulating drinks in the evening

3. And try breathing skills ideas

4. Timing of last meal in the day

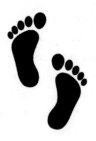

Footstep 8:

Healthy eating, managing relationships and coping with work

1. Healthy eating

Eating well and having a normal-range weight helps you to build better health and so cope better with pain. Being overweight can get you down. At least 50 per cent of people with pain are overweight. Key tips from people with pain are:

- **Do not** do another weight reduction diet . . . it can make you feel low even thinking about it!!

- Medications for pain and health problems often help put weight on. This is unhelpful and makes managing pain trickier. So explore options including healthy food choices and medication reviews with your doctor or pharmacist.

- Try and go Mediterranean instead!! So eat more healthy food like pasta, fish, lentils, chicken, vegetables and fruits, as these help joints, muscles and nerves work better. Use olive oil as your main cooking oil as it is a healthy oil. Explore more about these foods, known as the Mediterranean diet, on www.nhs.uk.

- Healthy eating helps you to lose weight and reduces your risk of heart disease, stroke, dementia, cancer and constipation, as well as depression and anxiety.

- Vitamin D is linked to persistent pain and it seems sensible to take daily supplements as often levels can be low in people with pain. Sunlight helps your body produce Vitamin D. Getting enough is difficult in winter or if you stay indoors a lot for other reasons – including pain. There are very few food sources of Vitamin D, other than oily fish and egg yolks. Check with your clinical team and explore NHS Choices to discover more.

- Never skip breakfast, as this helps the body be less stressed, tired – and painful! Start with *easy, small portions* like two or three tablespoons of cereal or yoghurt or half a banana. People with pain who skip breakfast find eating very small portions is a good start to eating better.

Fruit juices and water are healthy too and help reduce drinks with caffeine like coffee and tea.

• Eat regular meals with small portions if you are quite inactive. Snacks can be tempting but unhelpful for managing weight and pain!

Janice's breakfast

Janice hated breakfast, especially if she had been up at night with her neck nerve pains. So she just had a mug or two of coffee. Then the side effects of pain medications meant she skipped lunch. Late afternoon she had some biscuits and a banana and felt very full.

When she tracked her eating patterns she found she ate too much sweet food, often ate just once a day and felt really tired.

She set a goal to eat breakfast, just two tablespoons of muesli and one tablespoon of yoghurt. She ate breakfast most days and within two weeks she found she ate more and was less tired and grumpy. Her next goal was to have soup at lunchtime and continue her small breakfast. This helped her daily routine and she had more energy, better concentration and it helped her fitness plans. Three months on, 'I have lost 10 lbs just through having smaller portions and eating better . . . it feels good'.

Weight loss happens as fitness grows, with regular eating patterns and healthier food choices.

2. Managing relationships – connecting better with others

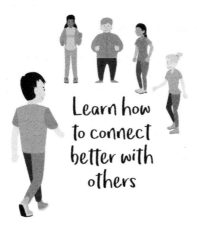

Learn how to connect better with others

Talking and sharing can feel like the last thing possible when pain dominates life. It's much easier to share or talk with your partner, family, friends or colleagues when you're in less pain and feel less stressed or low.

Anousha and her family

Anousha hated talking about her body pains. Her family could never work out what was going on except she was very quiet or just went to bed for hours. It made it tricky for the children and her husband Anil who worked as a taxi driver. It seemed things were stuck and Anousha just wanted it all to go away. Her sister Ama asked how the family could help her. They felt frustrated and concerned and it was difficult to plan and do things together. Anousha admitted she was fed up too and worried how to manage pain and family activities. Ama and she agreed that Anousha would:

- *Work on her goal to do a walk in the park twice a week.*

- *Share her plans for the day with the family and Anil and ask for their ideas for support.*

Her children said they would make her tea when she got back from the walk in the park. On 'bad pain days', Anousha would ask for help with cleaning and doing the meals to help her pace the day well. The family also came up with the idea that on very bad days they would organise a takeaway meal. Anousha felt more confident in her plans as the family helped out more with

> *chores. She shared with them her goal progress and, by pacing better, she was able to make two lovely family evening meals. The family loved her home cooking. She was thrilled and the family did their best to help on other nights!*

It can help to let people know how the pain limits you. Other people can't see the invisible effects of pain. Work with them on ways they can support your goals or help you live better with pain.

Help with relationship difficulties

Difficulties with partners and family members may need help and there are resources to explore at the end of this book. Sometimes young people caring for you, when the pain is disabling, can be supported with local young carer schemes.

3. Staying at or returning to work

The good news is that the skills in managing life with pain and being more confident turn out to be helpful:

* To stay at work or return to work

* To start studying or retraining

- For exploring other options like fostering or volunteering

- To develop new roles or activities in life

People find being in work a good experience in many ways, including helping routines and getting to know more people. They found they coped well with some difficult times on their route back to work or study. New coping skills used to manage pain helped work and other roles, especially pacing the work load and managing moods, like frustration (see Footstep 6).

Some tips:

- Think what needs to happen for you to return to or stay at work.

- Be flexible on what work you might do and where; volunteering lets you explore new possibilities of work areas.

- Ask for a phased return to work, as people do return this way successfully. Starting with just two–three hours per day for the first week and steadily building up work time has helped many people back to work.

- Be prepared to accept any support that is

offered at work, such as occupational health and retraining programmes or adaptations or aids like a desk where you can stand and sit, so pacing positions.

• Get your physiotherapist or GP on board to support you.

John's story

John went to a local community college due to work and sickness benefits pressures; he had to do something! He really struggled with reading and writing at school. He was left with little choice and took the plunge. The college was good fun and helpful. He discovered other people like him were also finding out what they could do through job skills training and experience, like business studies, running a shop, learning upholstery or electrical maintenance. He did some diploma courses and was thrilled to pass them. He found work within two months after a college work placement in a garden centre, as assistant manager. He realised he had struggled too long before taking the plunge: 'Do not wait – give training or new work a try and get good advice.'

Many people have taken control of their pain by choosing different Footsteps skills and resources. Some have started new jobs or careers, started businesses or hobbies and found valuable roles from volunteering to raise money for charities.

My action plan

What will help me to . . . ?

1. Eat healthily

2. Share with or get support from others

3. Manage a work plan

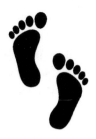

Footstep 9:

Relaxation and mindfulness: Soothe the body and mind

People with pain find that unwinding the body and mind makes a positive difference to their lives and their pain. Relaxation and mindfulness practice help to lessen pain levels, reduce tension and stress in both the body and mind and improve concentration. This is good news as these are key skills to living well with pain.

Of course, these skills require persistence and patience. Just like learning to play a musical instrument or learning to swim or cycle, practice is really vital. This isn't always easy. Pain can get in the way, for example being woken from sleep with a restless, painful body at 3 a.m. Other pressures in life can make it difficult to relax, like facing a difficult meeting with the boss about work. So it's important to be kind and patient when building relaxation and mindfulness skills. Try to practise regularly and accept that you may have days with no practice or occasional setbacks. It all leads to success and a valuable habit.

What is relaxation?

Relaxation happens when you guide (or someone else guides) the mind to unwind the tension and tightness within the body. It involves breathing skills and focusing the mind on relaxing images, colours or experiences. It also uses gentle movements where you tighten or stretch and relax with a focus on your breath to lessen the tension within the muscles and body. Most people who have struggled with pain say that it is so important to learn relaxation. It helps to do it with support and to keep doing it on good and bad days with pain.

Relaxation is also about helping you to unwind, like reading an enjoyable magazine, listening to relaxing music, fishing, potting plants or doing word puzzles.

Learning relaxation can be easier than you expect and many people say they can feel positive results very quickly.

'Learning and practising the diaphragmatic breathing helps a lot with soothing and calming me.'

'Safe place relaxation – keeps me calm and my energy levels recharge.'

It is about finding out when, where and how are the best ways to relax for you. The resources suggested at the end of this book are a practical guide to grow these skills.

What types of relaxation skills are there?

1. Breathing and muscle relaxation

- Belly breathing (also called diaphragmatic breathing)

- Progressive muscle relaxation

- On-the-spot arousal (anxiety or anger) reduction (OTSAR) see Appendix 2.

Explore the resources to help you start relaxation in practical ways.

2. Distract the mind's attention to imagine pleasurable activity like a walk in the countryside or along a beach and so shift focus away from pain and other unpleasant feelings.

3. Choosing activities that can help relax and unwind

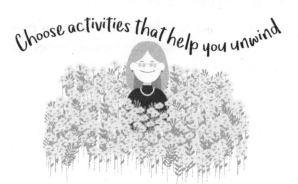

Choose activities that help you unwind

Some ideas to try and use often:

- Gentle exercise programmes like yoga, tai chi or Pilates

- Sitting in a beautiful garden and smelling the flowers

- Listening to a relaxation CD or app

- Listening to a favourite piece of music

- Taking a photograph of a beautiful scene

- Attending a local relaxation group, local gym or local self-help group

- Listening to recordings of nature like the sound on a sea shore or birds singing

- Knitting or crocheting

- A warm bath and using scented oils

Experiment and build your own relaxation programme. Choose to do one or even two things that are helpful each day.

A discovery of relaxation: Jacky and Dave's story

Jacky was in a mega struggle with stress, bill payment problems and the worst of pain flare-ups. Her friend Dave had pain too and had done a self-management course for pain where he found out about relaxation. He lent Jacky his course notes and a CD with some relaxation tracks, saying, 'Give it a go. It really helps; don't do all the tracks at once. Choose one track and explore it.' That night, to help her sleep, she chose to follow the relaxed muscle breathing track from the CD. She was drifting off when her mobile phone rang. It was her son and he would be late home. She felt irritated as she was feeling quite soothed and comfortable. She listened again to the same track and she slept through her son's arrival home at 1.00 a.m.

> *She woke once more, turned over and fell quickly back to sleep. She had a sense she was more rested in the morning. Dave rang that day to find out how she had got on. He was glad to hear that Jacky had a better night. He suggested that she explore more of the CD and use the guide to relaxation skills sheet. He shared, 'Find your two or three best tracks and work with them for a few weeks. I use the breathing one at work. No one notices and it gets me through the busy times on the job.'*

What is mindfulness?

Mindfulness is being aware of your body and mind in the 'now'. It is about noticing what you think, feel or want at this moment without engaging with the experience or being critical or judging yourself. It is exploring with all your senses – taste, touch, sound, sight and smell – and guides you to see your thoughts as events in the mind rather than facts or truths. It allows you to choose how to respond to your thoughts rather than react to them. It helps you make kinder choices on how to manage your pain, your situation or your thoughts.

Why is mindfulness helpful?

We now know that mindfulness helps us to live better with difficult health problems like pain, tiredness and so on. It also helps the brain to work better in many different ways, like improving memory or helping with attention so you focus and concentrate better. It is good for learning problem-solving and being creative, so helps self-management. Mindfulness practice helps to reduce stress hormones and lessen moods like anxiety, depression or anger and our thinking patterns that get tied in with them.

Stanter's experience

Mindfulness and meditation are about being mentally focused on the present moment, not absorbed in regrets, plans, worries or other thoughts. When we practise mindfulness we are more aware of the things that help us to be calm and happy and the thought patterns that take us in the opposite direction. With this awareness, we can take positive choices in everyday life.

It seems from recent scientific research that relaxed breathing and mindfulness help the nervous system to be soothed and less over-reactive and tense. This is really helpful for people living with pain as pain is seen by the brain as a threat, and it responds by turning up adrenaline levels in the body. Mindfulness (and relaxation too) help as they release soothing chemicals. These chemicals reduce adrenaline and other unhelpful chemicals that actually wind up your pain systems, making them more sensitive. Put another way, using mindfulness gives a safe and helpful natural tranquilliser. It helps taking steps towards acceptance and over time it can lessen the suffering due to pain itself. It supports you to learn the skills to live well with pain.

Like any other skill, mindfulness needs daily practice and guidance to use confidently. Just as people with diabetes need to manage their condition by using insulin every day and making changes to their eating habits and lifestyle, so people with pain discover the value of self-soothing through relaxation and mindfulness, positive self-talk and pacing activities. Mindfulness is something very simple to grasp but can be quite difficult to do, so let's explore Jan's moments to understand further.

Jan's 'moments' of mindfulness

www.painsupport.co.uk

It was a wet, cold day and I was not keen to do my regular walk. I'd had a bad night with back pain and a busy morning. I knew from experience that if I missed my walk and I stayed sitting or lying down my pain would be worse.

Somehow I found the energy to put on my wet weather gear and stepped out into the stormy day.

Soon I became recharged as I splashed through puddles and was whirled along by the wind. I started to take a real interest in all around me. I noticed the catkins dancing and pussy willows softly gleaming in the rain. My path led across a field where gulls and crows were feeding. They let out great squawks of annoyance at being disturbed as they took to the air. The gulls whirled round in the wind before settling down again. The rooks tried to fly in a straight line to a tall tree, the wind forcing them into zigzag patterns against the sky.

I love to watch birds, so I waited as they settled down on the field to feed again. Time stood still. Then I realised I had been standing for too long so headed for home. As I went indoors I noticed my pain was less and I felt boosted and re-energised.

How can I learn mindfulness and relaxation skills?

There are lots of ways to learn. It just depends on how you learn best. You could:

* Get support from a friend or help from a mindfulness trainer.

* Access an internet course, read a guide book or work with a CD course.

* Join a local relaxation class or mindfulness meditation course and practise at home.

There are mindfulness movement courses that link breathing and movement together and are very helpful for stiff and tight muscles and bodies.

At the end of this book there are ideas and resources that you can explore. Give them a try and if you are struggling then find some professional help. You could get support from a pain specialist physiotherapist, a talking therapist or a mindfulness teacher who can guide your relaxation and mindfulness skills.

Action plan

Ways to start relaxation and/or mindfulness practice. Be willing to experiment like Jacky did and explore resources.

Some ideas to help your plan start:

1. What relaxation and/or mindfulness can I include in my routines this week?

2. What could I use to help: CDs, Web-based resources?

3. How many minutes should I put aside for my practice?

4. When shall I do it? (Give a time in my day.)

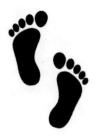

Footstep 10:

Managing setbacks

Setbacks are very common in managing pain. Being confident to deal with them is a *'must have'* skill for an easier time. Setbacks can be due to many reasons and sometimes just happen, just as they might for athletes in training. For athletes, it can be a setback due to injury, tiredness or mental or life challenges. A setback with pain is similar and often linked to tiredness, pacing difficulties, mood issues or medication changes, but sometimes for no obvious reason.

Sassia's story

Sassia's life wasn't getting any easier — sometimes she was in so much pain walking home the short distance from town that she would just sit on a

> *wall and cry. She would have to call her husband to collect her yet again!*
>
> *She had pain setbacks most months like clock-work. On those days walking up a flight of stairs felt like completing a marathon. Her pains in her shoulder, elbow, back and hips were excruciating in a setback. Now she predicted at least four or more setbacks a month and was puzzling on how she should manage them.*

Sassia is struggling to get to grips with the pain circle that traps her with pain setbacks. She realises that dealing with them is crucial.

Ways to manage setbacks

A setback plan helps you to cope with setbacks better and reduces the stress, sometimes panic, or low mood that they cause. Pete Moore shares his setback plan ideas below:

1. Ease back, easy does it

- Cut back on normal activities for some days. Take more, small regular BREAKS in the day, lie or sit down and unwind the body using re-laxation breathing.

- Bed rest weakens muscle strength rapidly. You lose about 1 per cent of total muscle strength each day if you totally rest up. So keep gently ACTIVE and moving to speed recovery and shorten setbacks.

- Be kind to yourself. Say 'NO' to any big, stressful or unhelpful demands until you feel stronger and more confident.

- Don't be too proud or scared to ASK for help from others, support helps in setbacks!

2. Pace more and keep active (see Footstep 3)

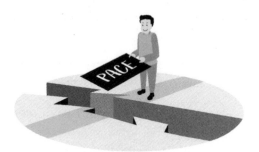

Setback?
Pace more and
keep active

- Remember: pace yourself even more. Begin gentle stretching and movement as soon as possible to regain flexibility. Start on the same day as the setback if possible! Your body will work *with you* if you take it gently, steadily and move often.

- Build up the time you spend stretching and moving. Keeping active may seem alien but don't be put off as it really does work!

- Use the effort scale to guide activities and fitness and choose effort levels 3–5 as you manage difficult days.

3. Relaxation

- Practise relaxation/s or mindfulness breathing . Explore Footstep 9.

- Do things to soothe and calm you: listening to music, knitting, doodling, stroking the cat or dog.

4. Refocus thinking

- Tackle your thoughts. Try not to think of the setback as the '*worst thing that can happen*'. This puts your mind and the pain into a negative spiral of thought and moods.

- Accept that you have a setback and now is the time for the plan. Share with yourself '*that just as it came, it will settle more easily. I now have a plan to help me get back on track.'* (See Footstep 1)

- Change your setback plan as you learn what helps your setbacks to be shorter and less severe.

Examples of a setback plan

Sassia's setback plan

- *Shop twice a week instead of once, pace two small trips to local shops, not one big super-market trip.*

- *Use my belly breathing with my stretches before going shopping.*

- *Cut down my stretch routine by 50 per cent for the next few days.*

- *Nice things to do: watch my favourite film; relax in a hot bath with scented oils.*

- *Plan some things to do when the setback has gone – my reward is 'a fun day trip soon'!*

Pete's plans

In my setbacks in the past, I would end up lying on the floor, resting up all day and then seeing the doctor again. Now I feel more confident in managing them and I actually go to the gym instead! I found staying active, gently stretching and exercising surprised me at first and I got through my setbacks much quicker.

Here's what helps me . . . now:

- *I am nice to myself and take it steady — 'easy does it days'.*

- *I tell myself: 'The setback has come, it will go.'*

- *I cut down all activities by about half the amount for a few days.*

- *I am kind to myself and give myself a treat. 'It is something to look forward to in a setback.'*

Preventing setbacks

Some handy tips to help you avoid having a setback or reduce them happening:

1. Prioritise and pace everyday jobs or work.

2. Break up tasks into smaller portions with effort level balanced. Watch for 'must-do' thinking – '*All this must get done, the pain is down and I should work on something*'. This is a **red alert** for a setback to kick in. (See Footstep 3.)

3. Shift your thinking and say to yourself, 'I can get this bit done today, I might get that done next week and I don't need to do that at all – someone else can do it.'

4. Keep your body gently fit and stretched every day as more fitness means fewer setbacks.

5. Help your body and mind, use relaxation practices with your focus on your breathing. (See Footstep 9.)

6. Explore and revisit often the ten keys to happier living.

GREAT DREAM
Ten keys to happier living

GIVING — Do things for others

RELATING — Connect with people

EXERCISING — Take care of your body

AWARENESS — Live life mindfully

TRYING OUT — Keep learning new things

DIRECTION — Have goals to look forward to

RESILIENCE — Find ways to bounce back

EMOTIONS — Look for what's good

ACCEPTANCE — Be comfortable with who you are

MEANING — Be part of something bigger

ACTION FOR HAPPINESS

www.actionforhappiness.org

My action plan for setbacks

Setback plans help keep your life on track, so explore the resources to guide your plans.

1. What changes can I make to prevent a setback?

2. Which activities shall I reduce (but not stop altogether) in a setback?

3. What stretches shall I do every day?

4. What rewards will keep me motivated?

Appendices

Appendix 1

Jen's goal ladder: her eight-week goal; each step is an action plan.

Jen's Goal Ladder example to guide SMART goal plans

	Things that help my progress	Goal: to create a new flower bed	Things that block my progress
Week 7	Nick, my partner, made a cup of tea and said 'a great achievement'. Lucky the flower bed is three feet off the ground so less bending down.	Walk X 25mins + stretches X 3 daily. Add mindfulness breathing. Plant + water in small shrubs – ask Nick to dig bigger holes. Remember: half-fill watering can!	Some plants dried out – I forgot to water them. Shrubs heavier than I thought.
Weeks 5–6	My reward: bunches of tulips – lovely yellow ones. Plants arrived; needed water. Patience and pacing – don't overdo it again!!	Walk 15 mins + daily stretches due to setback. Reset effort at 5/6. Use iPod relaxation track as a break. Water new plants, put into 'my' new bed! Finish plant cutting.	Bad pain in week 5 – *effort level* 9, so reduced it – 6/10.
Week 4	Found playing music very helpful when weeding. A stool helped pacing. Started choosing the plants to go in – excited.	Walk 25 mins + stretches X 2 daily. Muscle stretches with breathing. Weed more deep-rooted plants. Only half-fill bucket to lift into compost bin.	Needed Nick to move compost bags – tried and failed myself; filled them too much. New plan needed here.
Week 2	Noticed my pacing was helping progress. Explored planting ideas with friends. Effort level 5 – ? bit easy.	Help bend better, so stretches X 2 daily. Use relaxed breathing. Weed 10 mins; half-fill bucket. Start walking goal.	Handle broken – needed new bucket.
Start	Made a plan so know where to begin.	Choose tools + buckets. Plan areas to weed in 10ft-square bed in four weeks. Do X3 arm & neck stretches before gardening.	Neck very stiff. Rushed too quickly at the weeding.

Appendix 1. My goal ladder for my ...... week goal, with action plan for each step (see Footstep 4)

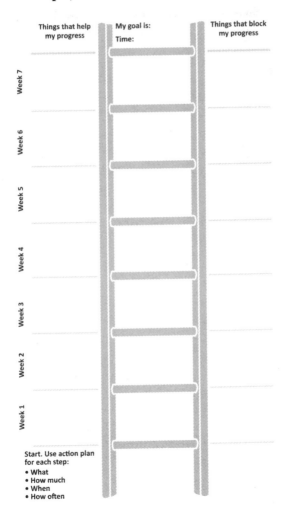

Appendix 2

On The Spot Anxiety (or Anger) Reduction

OTSAR is a breathing skill that is specifically helpful with feelings of anxiety or anger where the body is aroused by the release of adrenaline.

If you experience such feelings, this exercise will help you to breathe them away once you notice the warning signs of these feelings or thoughts.

Preparation

Get into a comfortable sitting or lying position.

Place a hand on your chest and a hand on your belly just above the waistline. Breathe OUT slowly and steadily to empty your lungs. You should notice the hand on your belly moves in as the air leaves your lungs.

Breathe in and notice the hand on your belly moves *out*. If the hand on your belly does not move and the hand on your chest does then you are only breathing from the upper part of your lungs. It is important that you experiment and breathe in and out to make certain you are using all the lung space and diaphragm in this skill.

Step 1: Plonk yourself in a chair and feel held and supported by it. Breathe OUT – blow away the anger through your mouth (it is very easy to breathe in first, so practise just straight breaths out)

Step 2 Breathe IN through the nose to a count of four

Step 3 Breathe OUT to a count of six

Continue for *at least four minutes* or longer. This approach switches on the body chemicals that block adrenaline release and therefore calms the body and mind.

People with pain have found this one of the most helpful skills for lots of situations where they feel anxious or angry, or their pain makes them stressed.

Resources

Websites

www.actionforhappiness.org

www.bigwhitewall.com – Big White Wall; online supportive community to help deal with moods.

www.britishpainsociety.org.uk – Explore the 'People living with pain' area and leaflets on medications and treatments.

www.healthtalkonline.org; useful resource about people with pain.

www.nhs.uk/Livewell/Goodfood/Pages/what-is-a-Mediterranean-diet.aspx – good guide to changing foods and ways to healthier eating.

www.painassociationscotland.com

www.painconcern.org.uk – See videos: what-is-self-management.

www.paintoolkit.org – booklets in 25 languages.

www.patient.info – Good resource on the range of pain medications.

www.rcoa.ac.uk/faculty-of-pain-medicine/opioids-aware – Up-to-date resource on using opioids.

www.relate.org.uk – Valuable site to access practical help for relationship issues.

www.sheffieldpersistentpain.com – Goal-setting pacing and setback videos, information from people with pain. Also leaflets like 'Explain Pain' and about medications, with ways to use them well.

www.happify.com – Shares how the brain works and some interesting (sometimes fun) ways to help change thinking and behaviours or habits.

www.mind.org.uk – MIND provides valuable resources and has local support services in many places. It has courses on relaxation, mindfulness and coping with moods and, in some places, pain.

For CBT-based booklets and audio resources on sleep:

www.ntw.nhs.uk/pic/selfhelp – Excellent range of sleep and mood resources, like depression, anxiety, panic and anger.

www.sleepio.com – International sleep expert Professor Espie shares an online programme to help you sleep well.

www.nhs.uk/pages/home.aspx – Information on sleep apnoea.

www.overcoming.co.uk – CBT-based self-help books on a range of physical and mental health problems.

Mindfulness:

www.breathworks-mindfulness.co.uk – Invaluable resource for courses and a range of CDs, books, etc.

www.soundstrue.com – Useful resources online from mindfulness practitioners.

www.stitchlinks.com – Focus on knitting to help manage pain mindfully.

www.youtube.com/watch?v=gQfKpPpOxBM – 'Mindfulness for Life' by Mark Williams.

www.youtube.com/watch?v=iSGsTWcofhM – 'How mindfulness can help cope with pain'; Vidayamala Burch

www.youtube.com/watch?v=rUMF5R7DoOA – 'Self-compassion' by Dr Kristin Neff.

www.youtube.com/watch?v=x_DgOoKrkDA – Ruby Wax on mindfulness.

Books

Living Beyond your Pain – Using Acceptance and Commitment Therapy to Ease Chronic Pain, J. Dahl (2006), ISBN 978-1572244092, New Harbinger.

Overcoming Chronic Pain, Cole et al (2004), ISBN 9781841199702, Robinson.

Overcoming Sleep Problems, Colin Espie, www.overcoming.co.uk, ISBN 9781845290702.

The Mindfulness Journal, Corinne Sweet (2014), ISBN 9780752265605, Boxtree.

The Pain Management Plan, R. Lewin (2010), ISBN 9780956662804, Npowered Ltd.

The Sleep Book, Guy Meadows, www.orionbooks.co.uk, ISBN 978140915761-8.

Books with CDs:

Mindfulness for Health, Vidyamala Burch & Danny Penman (2013), ISBN 9780749959241, Piatkus.

You Are Not Your Pain, Vidayamala Burch and Danny Penman (2015), ISBN 9781250052674, Flatiron.

The Pain Management Plan, R. Lewin, ISBN 9780956662804, Npowered Ltd.

Videos

Three key videos that explain pain and the brain very well and in different languages:

1. https://www.youtube.com/watch?v=C_3ph B93rvI 'Understanding pain in five minutes' is invaluable to make sense of persistent pain.

2. www.youtube.com/watch?v=I7wfDenj6CQ&s ns=em 'How does your brain respond to pain' by Karen Davies.

3. www.youtube.com/watch?v=gwd-wLdIHjs
   'Why things hurt' by Lorimer Moseley, TedX
   talk Adelaide.

www.painassociationscotland/videos/goalsetting.

www.paincd.org – Helpful audio resources on managing pain.

Health apps

www.ntw.nhs.uk/pic/selfhelp – All twenty-three CBT leaflets are an app for tablet/smartphone.

www.painsense.co.uk – Pain Toolkit app and Pain Plan app.